What Can I Eat?

A Guide to Nutrition
After Gastric Bypass

What Can I Eat?

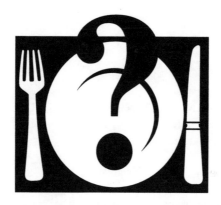

A Guide to Nutrition After Gastric Bypass

By Arlene Swantko, R.D., L.D.

NUTRITION TECHNIQUES, LLC, Columbia, Maryland

PUBLISHED BY NUTRITION TECHNIQUES, LLC
9459 Vollmerhausen Drive
Columbia, Maryland 21046

Library of Congress Catalog Card Number has been applied for

ISBN 0-9759714-0-9

PRINTED IN THE UNITED STATES OF AMERICA

This book is dedicated to my husband, Russ, for his continuous support and encouragement, and to my daughters, Amy and Jessie, who are my greatest accomplishment.

Acknowledgments

This book would not have been possible without the help of my editor, Joan Waclawski. Her quest for perfection and professional results have made this project an experience that has been challenging, rewarding, and pleasant. With every stage of the process, she has always been positive, encouraging, and realistic. Her editing skills, inquisitiveness, and attention to detail made this book the best that it could be.

Dr. Kuldeep Singh and Dr. Andrew Averbach have always had confidence and trust in me to be the source of nutritional guidance for all of their gastric bypass patients. Their technical skills and medical knowledge are awe-inspiring. The respectful manner in which they deal with their patients and other professionals is gratifying.

Cathy Carr-Younger, R.N., has been my major source of knowledge about gastric bypass surgery. Over the years, she has become a friend as well. Together we celebrate the successes of our patients and try to encourage them to deal with the challenges they encounter. We share both our victories and our frustrations. I value her opinion and advice and know that she is always available to hear me out.

Bea Flynn teaches me something whenever I talk to her. Her insight and knowledge about the psychological impact of obesity on an individual's life has been enlightening. She puts into perspective why people act and react as they do before and after gastric bypass. Everything she does is with a great deal of compassion and understanding of the complex nature of all of us.

And finally, I owe a debt of gratitude to all of the hundreds of gastric bypass patients who have allowed me to instruct them about the importance of proper nutrition after gastric bypass. I have learned a tremendous amount about the process from them. They have shared some of their most embarrassing and poignant moments with me. I have calmed them down and lifted them up. I have been stern about my requirements and rigid with some of my recommendations. They all know that I have high expectations for them and that I want them to be successful with gastric bypass many years into the future. I could not have written this book without them and their experiences.

Table of Contents

Acknowledgments i

Introduction 1

Chapter 1: How Much Do You Know About Gastric Bypass? 5

Chapter 2: Now That You've Made the Decision 17

Chapter 3: Transition Period Immediately After Surgery 21

Chapter 4: Eating After Gastric Bypass 25

Chapter 5: Vitamin, Mineral, and Protein Supplementation 31

Chapter 6: Two-Week Follow-Up Visit 37

Chapter 7: Making Lifestyle Changes More Permanent 45

Chapter 8: Emotional & Psychological Aspects
of Eating Differently 51

Chapter 9: There Is Life After Gastric Bypass Surgery 61

Appendix: Frequently Asked Questions 63

Suggested Resources 69

I feel like a butterfly coming out of my cocoon

I finally see the beauty from within

I spread my wings

I soar

Light as a feather

— Patricia Z.

Introduction

When I received a phone call from Kuldeep Singh, M.D., one Monday in February 2001, I had no idea that I would become involved with a procedure that would be a life-changing event for hundreds of people. Dr. Singh asked me if I would meet with him to discuss gastric bypass surgery, or GBS, a new procedure he was planning to add to his already advanced laparoscopic surgery practice at St. Agnes Hospital in Baltimore, Maryland. If he could assemble a team of practitioners to work with the procedure, he was ready to move forward.

My involvement would be to educate the patients before the surgery, to explain the types of foods they would be allowed to eat afterwards, and to emphasize the importance of good nutrition for the rest of their lives. It seemed easy enough, since I had been a registered dietitian for over 20 years and had counseled hundreds of patients on the importance of good nutrition. It would be my responsibility to learn all that I could in the coming months about gastric bypass surgery and to design the teaching materials to use with the patients.

I am always ready to learn new things and to accept a challenge. There was not a lot of literature available about the gastric bypass eating protocol, but I read whatever I could find. The coordinator of the program, Cathy Carr-Younger, R.N., who had had gastric bypass surgery, became my major source of information about the procedure. Her first-hand knowledge and experience with the surgery proved to be the best method for me to learn which specific details I needed to convey to the patients.

As I began to work with the candidates for GBS, I came to realize that the surgery could produce phenomenal results if the individual made a serious commitment to lifestyle changes. For many patients, the surgery would mean an end to diabetes, high blood pressure, and joint pain. The fact that they would be able to lead a happier and healthier life would make the choice to have the surgery the most important decision most of them had ever made.

The success of our patients with gastric bypass surgery has been unbelievable from the standpoint of significant weight loss, improved health, self-esteem, and quality of life. It has made such dramatic differences in the lives of so many people that I am constantly amazed at the fact that I have been involved in their education and adjustment to a new life. Working with over 500 patients has also shown me that gastric bypass is not the right choice for everyone. Changing the way one thinks about and reacts to food is a tremendous task and the ultimate challenge for gastric bypass patients. Their body has been altered to accept only small amounts of food; however, their mindset has to be altered as well.

While much more has been published about the surgery within the last two years, the Internet is exploding with information, and television programs describing the surgery are broadcast regularly, there seems to be a need for more education about life after GBS. Many of my patients have said to me that there is no way to explain or describe the emotional reaction to making extreme changes to the food you eat. It is very hard for me to convey to people the impact that the decision to have gastric bypass will have on their lives.

The idea for this book evolved after hearing the stories of so many people and knowing that their advice to others contemplating the surgery could have a profound effect on the decision. Perhaps it would make someone realize that the surgery is not for him. Or, it could help someone realize that she is not alone with her feelings and emotions after the surgery. I asked over 100 patients of mine who have had GBS to fill out a questionnaire and to give me their honest opinions about the decision-making process, the outcome, their lives afterwards, and any negative aspects the surgery has presented to them. The quotes in this book are taken directly from their responses to this questionnaire. None of them have been edited or altered; for privacy's sake, only the first name and last initial of the individuals are used.

It has been extremely gratifying to work with this patient population. For many of the men and women I have counseled, the fact that there was a procedure that could be performed to enable them to lose a significant amount of weight gave them hope for the first time in their lives. The success of these men and women has encouraged me to write this book in order to describe to others the new life that is possible after gastric bypass.

1

How Much Do You Know About Gastric Bypass?

According to the National Institutes of Health Clinical Guidelines (1998), "Gastrointestinal surgery (gastric restriction) or gastric bypass (Roux-en-Y) can result in substantial weight loss, and therefore is an available weight loss option for well-informed and motivated patients with BMI > 40 or BMI < 35, who have comorbid conditions and acceptable operative risks."

Body Mass Index (BMI) is a relationship between weight and height that is associated with body fat and health risk. Comorbid conditions refers to illnesses and disabling conditions associated with severe obesity, such as diabetes, arthritis, hypertension, urinary incontinence, sleep apnea, reflux, and shortness of breath. There must be evidence to prove that all efforts to lose weight through traditional means have been exhausted before surgery is considered as an option.

The Gastric Bypass Procedure

Gastrointestinal surgery for obesity, also called bariatric (dealing with the causes, prevention, and treatment of obesity) surgery, alters the digestive process. The operation results in weight loss by closing off parts of the stomach to make it smaller. Operations that only reduce the size of the stomach are called *restrictive* operations because they restrict the amount of food that the stomach can contain. There are also operations that combine stomach restriction with a partial bypass of the small intestine. These procedures create a direct connection from the stomach to the lower segment of the small intestine, thereby bypassing some portions of the digestive tract that absorb calories and nutrients. These are known as *malabsorptive* procedures.

Is there a single defining moment or experience that made you decide to have GBS?

Quote from Lisa V.:
"My life had become so out of control, I was only dealing with the stress by overeating. Things really came to a boiling point and my health was rapidly failing. I was no longer able to do so many things. I looked terrible and was unrecognizable at 400 lbs. to some people that I've known my whole life. I was experiencing so much physical, emotional, spiritual, and mental pain that my daily life was truly unbearable. I was experiencing fear and anxiety because of all of this. Also, though I had decided to do the surgery, my mother was not convinced that it was a good idea. I bought tickets for my mom and I to go to a concert and I went through a lot of trouble to make sure that I had an end of aisle seat so that I could move the arm of the seat and would be able to fit in the seat. The tickets cost almost $300 and I had gotten them for my mother for Mother's Day 2002. When we arrived, I was horrified to see that the arm didn't move on the seat. I couldn't fit and I started to

cry in front of a lot of people. My mom and I were so devastated by this that the surgery was never again questioned and I had the surgery August 2002."

According to the American Society for Bariatric Surgery and the National Institutes of Health, Roux-en-Y gastric bypass is the current gold standard procedure for weight loss surgery. It is the most frequently performed procedure for weight loss in this country.

Roux-en-Y gastric bypass is a procedure in which a small pouch is created by stapling a portion of the stomach off to create a divide (see FIGURE 1). The remainder of the stomach is not removed. It will still secrete beneficial digestive fluids that are channeled into the small intestine. A Y-shaped section of the small intestine is attached to the pouch to allow food to bypass the lower stomach, the duodenum (the first segment of the small intestine), and the first portion of the jejunum (the second segment of the small intestine). This bypass reduces the amount of calories and nutrients the body can absorb. This procedure is usually done using a minimally invasive technique called laparoscopic surgery. When performing the surgery laparoscopically, the surgeon makes four or more small incisions in the abdomen through which slender surgical instruments are passed. This eliminates the need for a large incision and creates less tissue damage.

With Roux-en-Y gastric bypass, there is greater weight loss and long-term maintenance of weight loss than with the other

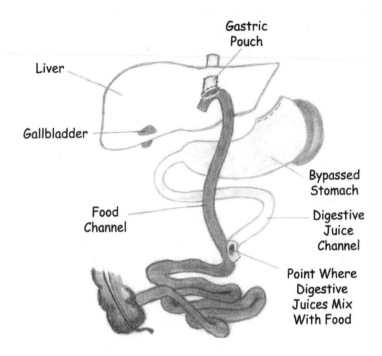

Liver

Gastric
Pouch

Gallbladder

Bypassed
Stomach

Food
Channel

Digestive
Juice
Channel

Point Where
Digestive
Juices Mix
With Food

Illustration by Jessie Swantko

FIGURE 1: Diagram of the Roux-en-Y Gastric Bypass

methods of GBS. Drawbacks of the surgery include potential sensitivity to volume and types of food consumed; high fat foods and high sugar foods may not be tolerated; and dehydration may result if inadequate fluids are consumed. Problem foods tend to be soft breads, pasta, rice, fried and fatty foods, and carbonated beverages.

Weight loss after GBS generally occurs for up to 18 months, with the most rapid loss occurring during the first six months. The surgery has an impact on disease risk, with studies showing a 90 percent postoperative reduction rate in obesity-related diseases. It can reverse diabetes, control hypertension, and improve physical mobility and quality of life. Gastric bypass is recognized by the medical profession as a method of treatment for Type II diabetes, since a high percentage of patients have normal glucose levels after the surgery.

Up to 20 percent of patients who have weight-loss surgery require follow-up operations to correct complications. Abdominal hernia is the most common complication reported. The increase in laparoscopic surgeries, which eliminate the large incision and minimize tissue damage, has helped to reduce the development of post-surgical hernias. However, patients who weigh more than 350 pounds or who have had previous abdominal surgery may not be good candidates for laparoscopy. Other less common complications include perforation or leakage of the stomach/intestine, spleen injury, blood clot in the lung, stoma stenosis (obstruction of the gastric outlet), and wound infection.

It must be mentioned that, in addition to the Roux-en-Y procedure, the Lap Band has been approved for use in weight loss surgery. It is an inflatable band that is placed around the upper stomach to create a small gastric pouch. This limits food consumption and creates an earlier feeling of fullness. The band is implanted laparoscopically and is then adjusted over time (either tightened or loosened) to meet individual patient needs. Once the band is in place, it is inflated with saline. Subsequent adjustments are made through a portal under the skin.

The Lap Band is intended to remain in place permanently, but it can be surgically removed, if necessary. People who get the Lap Band will need to diet and exercise in order to maintain their weight loss. The average weight loss is approximately 36 percent to 38 percent of excess weight, as measured two and three years after the surgery. Some patients manage to lose 100 percent of their excess weight; however, some do not lose any weight, and a few continue to gain weight. Side effects from the Lap Band include nausea and vomiting, heartburn, abdominal pain, and slippage or pouch enlargement. In studies done with patients who have had the Lap Band inserted, 25 percent have had the entire system removed, mostly because of adverse side effects. In about one-third of those patients, insufficient weight loss was also reported as a contributing factor to the decision to have it removed.

Most people who have bariatric surgery notice a marked difference in their appetites and hunger levels. It is often the case that cravings for certain foods diminish and foods that were once favorites are no longer appealing. It is thought that the procedure serves to decrease levels of the stomach hormone *ghrelin*, which controls both appetite and hunger. The lower levels of ghrelin may be responsible for making it easier to lose weight after gastric bypass than with traditional dieting methods. The reduced size of the stomach, of course, contributes significantly to the ability to be satisfied with a much smaller amount of food.

The combination of hormonal effects and reduced stomach size is what makes the surgery a successful method for weight loss. The fact that both appetite and hunger are more easily satisfied after gastric bypass makes significant weight loss more achievable. Bear in mind, however, that the surgery is a tool to assist the person in losing weight. It can bring a morbidly obese person to the point where eating properly and exercising will be effective and allow that person to lose more weight than ever before. The challenge is to permanently incorporate proper food choices and regular exercise into one's lifestyle. It is not a quick fix and will only work if the individual works at it and with it.

Before You Consider GBS

The individual should research the gastric bypass procedure thoroughly and obtain answers to any questions he or she may have. It is important to know that surgeons differ in their approach to the procedure. Some require gastric bypass candidates to lose weight before the surgery, either by traditional dieting or by using a liquid diet product. The skill level of the surgeon may determine whether the surgery will be done laparoscopically. Not all surgeons are capable of this method. Others who are skilled in the laparoscopic technique prefer it to minimize risk to the patient, although, again, patients weighing more than 350 pounds may not be good candidates for the laparoscopic procedure. You owe it to yourself to thoroughly research the surgeon and the level of experience and success rate of the practice before you have even an initial consultation. If you are in doubt about a surgeon you are considering, continue to interview other surgeons before making your final decision.

Communication with the surgeon's office staff regarding follow-up appointments and phone calls will be very important afterwards. If you have doubts about the level of assistance you get from the office prior to the surgery, take this into consideration when choosing the surgeon. If you have problems or concerns after the surgery, you will appreciate staff members who respond efficiently. Pay attention to your instincts; ask the surgeon about his successes and failures with the procedure. A surgeon who is not forthcoming with this information should be reconsidered. Get references. It is helpful to talk to others who have had the surgery performed by the same surgeons.

Not everyone is a good candidate for the surgery. A good surgeon should be able to determine at the initial visit whether he will be able to perform gastric bypass on the patient. For some individuals, their obesity may have progressed to a point at which they are at higher risk for complications after any surgery. If there are cardiac problems, stroke risks, circulation problems, or serious immobility issues, the surgery could create additional problems and even result in death.

The Internet has influenced the popularity of gastric bypass, probably more so than for any other surgical procedure. That fact is both good and bad. Some information obtained from the websites is positive, informative, professional, and accurate. However, personal testimonials and diaries found on the websites can have a negative effect on people and also give false information and impressions. It is essential that any information or advice taken from an individual's account be considered anecdotal until it has been verified by a professional.

The importance of having a psychological evaluation before gastric bypass cannot be overemphasized. It takes a professional who is familiar with the impact of the surgery to do a thorough and relevant assessment of the person who is contemplating it. Regardless of how prepared and informed the person seems to be, the psychological impact of having to change the way you eat is enormous. Immediately after the surgery, it is not unusual for the patient to feel blue, depressed, or sad. The question, "What have I done to myself?" can reverberate in the person's mind throughout the first days after surgery.

Having a strong support system is essential. A person who is suddenly thrown into a new lifestyle which excludes food needs caring, understanding, and patient people around him or her. At this point, some people realize that food has been their "best friend." True grieving can occur over the loss of this friend. This further complicates the recovery process, a time when emotions are already running high. For someone who has emotional or psychological issues, the additional stress can be devastating. A supportive environment after gastric bypass makes all the difference in adapting to a new way of living and eating.

The nutrition consultation prior to surgery is valuable for several reasons. Foremost, it enables the nutritionist/dietitian to explain the dietary changes the patient will be required to make, and the reasons for making the changes. It allows time for patients to have their own questions answered regarding food intake after surgery and to get acquainted with the dietitian who is going to play a major role in their adaptation to a new lifestyle. Most people realize that gastric bypass surgery will have a serious impact on their food choices and that they will have to give priority to their nutritional needs for the rest of their life. The consultation helps the dietitian to assess whether the individual is ready for the challenge the surgery will present. If the dietitian has any reservations about the patient's ability to follow the dietary requirements, the treatment team must be informed. It is not advisable to perform gastric bypass on anyone who does not comprehend or accept the nutritional requirements that will need to be followed.

It is helpful for the spouse, a family member, or a friend to also attend the consultation. There is a great deal of information conveyed and it is easy to miss something. The dietitian may also be able to determine at that point whether there is a strong level of support among family and friends for the surgery. It can be the case that the individual wants the surgery and the family is afraid of complications, or the family is pushing for the surgery and the patient is not ready for the commitment. A perceptive dietitian will notice these factors and report them to the team.

Please include any additional comments or observations you would like to make concerning GBS.

Quote from Kathie N:

"I think people are so misinformed about GBS surgery. They think you can eat anything and still lose weight. A GBS patient MUST be aware of all the misinformation out there. They need to be ready to 'defend' their choice, as there are 'those' who will tell you 'Oh, don't do it. You won't be able to eat anything and you'll never enjoy food again.' NOT TRUE! I still love food — I just make better choices now!

"The real truth is they don't want you to succeed — and it's because they are jealous of what you can become and what you can achieve. And, when you make your decision — one way or the other — hold true to your convictions. You are the ONLY one who can decide if this is for you — it is a 'way of life' that you MUST be willing to lead forever. Think of yourself first, you are the only one who cares the most about you! And, you are the only one who can change your life for the better ... forever!"

———————

Quote from Gail G.:

"Take into account your personality. I don't like to be told what to do. I prefer to choose what rules and regulations I obey. *Having* to follow a rigid, high protein diet makes me resentful. I feel that I am trapped and have little flexibility with my food choices."

The most successful gastric bypass programs include a great deal of education and information prior to the surgery. Many surgeons require their prospective patients to attend support groups and information sessions prior to their initial appointments. This surgery is in a category by itself with respect to the life-altering adjustments that will be necessary afterwards.

A good surgeon is going to perform gastric bypass flawlessly. The challenge to the patient is to commit to the changes that must be made in order to be successful. Gastric bypass surgery is not just a simple procedure that ends with the physical recovery of the patient. The nutritional, psychological, and emotional changes that are expected afterwards cannot be emphasized enough. Educating the patient about what changes to expect and emphasizing the need to deal with the changes as they are experienced is crucial to the individual's success.

2

Now That You've Made the Decision

The next phase in the process is submission of all of the medical information, consultation reports, and test results (gallbladder ultrasound, sleep study), if needed, to the insurance company. Insurance coverage for the procedure varies greatly. It is highly advised that, before you take the first step towards having gastric bypass surgery, you check with your health insurance carrier regarding coverage. Different insurance companies can have exclusion policies for the surgery and different requirements to qualify. For some, coverage is denied, appealed, and then approved. The insurance companies' policies differ from state to state, and from one company to another.

Some surgeons who perform bariatric surgery do not participate with any insurance companies. Financially, it may be impossible for most people to have the surgery if the procedure is not covered by their health insurance. For those who can afford the expense, however, it may be money well-spent, even if they have to pay for it themselves.

It typically takes several weeks or months to get approval and authorization for the surgery. This period of time can be very stressful. It is nerve-wracking, yet exciting, to feel that the chance for a normal life is nearly within your grasp. Use this time wisely. Think long and hard about your decision and the amount of change that will be required. Some may ultimately decide not to go through with gastric bypass. It is better to delay the surgery until you are 150 percent sure that you are ready to take on the challenge. Gastric bypass is not something you try out and then change if you do not like it. It is a choice to forever live within its restrictions.

The decision to have gastric bypass surgery can, in some ways, be compared to the decision to have a baby. As a prospective parent, you can read volumes about childbearing, child rearing, and parenting, feel as though you are well-prepared for the birth, and then, when the baby finally comes, find that it is a humbling experience to be responsible for a new life. The same can be said for the decision to have GBS. Until you are home from the hospital and relearning the most fundamental life skill — eating — you may never have felt so helpless. You may have felt that you were ready, but it can be very overwhelming to be intimidated by the task of eating. Making the final decision to have the surgery is not to be taken lightly. It is not something that you can give back or return. It is final, just like having a child.

Again, the support of family and friends during this preoperative period is most important. It is not unusual to doubt your decision and feel that you could be making a mistake. This is a good time to talk to others who have had the surgery and get their input. Doubts and concerns are common and it helps to know that others have experienced the same feelings.

What advice would you have to offer to friends and co-workers of those who have had GBS?

Quote from Barb M.:
"#1 Support your friend, be there!
#2 Attend support group meetings with them so you can better understand how to help them post surgery when they return to work.
#3 Don't be jealous of them, the only thing they have now that they didn't have before is a better quality of life and a new beginning at life! Embrace them, love them, and enjoy your new friend!"

In terms of health, it is not wise to throw caution to the wind and disregard your diet and medical concerns because you know you will soon have surgery to "fix" these issues. Diabetes could develop or worsen, cardiac issues may arise, and uncontrolled hypertension could lead to stroke. This is not the time to allow your health to deteriorate. Making dietary changes, doing some gentle exercise, drinking more water, and cutting down on sweets and sodas are great ways to prepare yourself for the surgery. During this time, some surgeons require that gastric bypass patients lose 10 percent of their weight before the surgery is performed. Also, some require a liquid diet for two weeks before the surgery to prepare your system for the transition.

It is on the agenda of some people to have a "Last Supper" before the surgery. If this is in your plans, do not do it right before the surgery. Eat lightly for two to three days before gastric bypass to allow the food to be digested and eliminated.

Describe your most positive experience with GBS.

Quote from Patricia A.:

"My most positive experience with GBS has been the entire team approach through the office of Dr. Singh and Averbach. Through every step of my journey someone has been available to answer questions and calm fears. I never felt when contacting a member of the team that I was being a nuisance or a bother. It seems crucial, to me, that this team approach be available. Having professionals — psychologist, nutritionist, nurse coordinator — on call at all times is most reassuring to those on the weight loss journey."

Any additional comments or observations you would like to make concerning GBS?

Quote from Donna B.:

"This surgery is not for everyone. It is a lifesaving 'tool' that will only work if you use it correctly. This is bariatric surgery, not brain surgery. If you have issues in your life that cause you to overeat, surgery will not cure them. You have to face those issues as well, or you will find yourself not using the tool correctly and gaining your weight back. I have seen it happen and it is sad to go through surgery and still not be able to control your food issues."

3

Transition Period Immediately After Surgery

Physically, recovery after laparoscopic gastric bypass is easier than if an open procedure was done. If the procedure was done laparoscopically, the stay in the hospital usually averages three to four days. The patient who has had gastric bypass performed with an open procedure may be hospitalized for at least five days.

Depending on the individual, there may be different reactions to the pain after surgery. It is not unusual for some people to experience very little pain after gastric bypass. There are others, however, who have serious pain. It is very much an individual issue and relates to the body's reaction to the surgery and the healing process. If the procedure was done laparoscopically, the pain and recovery process are generally not as long or difficult. With an open surgery, there is, naturally, a longer recovery period. In either case, driving a car is not allowed for a minimum of two weeks, nor is any heavy lifting allowed. It is wise to review the physical limitations with your surgeon upon discharge from the hospital. Those who do not follow the restrictions usually regret it. As with most things, common sense is important. This is yet another reason to have a support system, with others who can do things that you may not be permitted to do, like run errands, do laundry, and lift small children.

In the practice I am associated with, patients are discharged on liquids and puréed/blenderized foods. A completely liquid diet is not recommended. The gentle intake of smooth foods will help the anastomosis, or opening, from the pouch to the intestine heal. Foods that are merely cut into small pieces are not acceptable at this point.

This care regarding the texture of the foods is not prompted by a concern about choking, or of not being able to chew properly; it is matter of the food leaving the newly created stomach pouch gently and without pressure or discomfort. Thus, the food *must* be moist, soft, and the consistency of applesauce. Treat your "new little stomach" like a baby. The anastomosis is about the size of a dime. There are sutures around the opening which will heal; however, it is not a good idea to add stress to the area.

If foods are too thick, starchy, dry, or chunky, the opening may clog. People describe the sensation as feeling that the food is "stuck." If this is experienced, some people may feel that they have to make themselves vomit to remove the food; others can cough to dislodge it; or some may just wait for the food to move on its own. Drinking fluids usually will make matters worse, since the fluid will not be able to pass through the clogged opening but will just rest on top of the food, adding more pressure to the area. The feeling is not comfortable and few want to experience it again. The main point is to make certain that the food is moist and smooth before it goes into your mouth. After such an episode, some people are reluctant to eat again. This can be avoided if the food is consistently moist before you begin to eat it.

It is extremely helpful, and is usually required, for patients to keep an accurate food record after discharge, writing down everything they eat and drink each day, giving the time and approximate amount of food. The food record is the best tool to track problems, should they occur. Often, it is something simple that may be causing a problem, and the food record makes it easier to find. Time between meals can be a problem, as can the amount or texture of the food. With the food record, many times the individual can figure out what happened — for example, eating too much or too fast.

It is not unusual to be afraid to eat. Fear of vomiting or doing damage to the pouch is common. It is imperative to learn how to eat in a different way, and communication with the dietitian is critical if there are problems. The risk of becoming dehydrated is increased if adequate fluids are not consumed. The intake of fluids should take priority over eating, if a choice must be made.

The pouch is about the size of a jumbo egg, holding approximately 60 milliliters of fluid, or 2 ounces. The average, full-sized stomach holds about 1,500 milliliters of fluid, or 3 pints.

Patients are advised to eat 2 to 3 tablespoons of puréed food every three to four hours for the first two weeks. (This means while you are awake — you do not have to wake up during the night to eat.) The amount of food can vary from person to person; usually you are able to consume more as time passes. It is important to listen to your body for signs of fullness. If you feel full, stop eating. Even a small amount of extra food can make you feel uncomfortable and stuffed. The concept of "cleaning your plate" will quickly be forgotten. It is not a good idea to have someone else tell you how much you should eat. It is up to you to decide whether you have had enough and when you should stop. The best approach to take is to eat small amounts more frequently at first to prevent an uncomfortably full feeling.

After GBS, you cannot eat and drink at the same time. If there is fluid in the pouch and you begin to eat, you will feel full too soon. It is recommended that you stop drinking 20 to 30 minutes before you plan to eat. The fluids leave the pouch quickly. Then, it is empty to receive the food. After you have eaten, it is best to wait 20 to 30 minutes before you begin to drink again. Many people are concerned about this point, since they are very used to eating and drinking at the same time. If the food you are eating is moist, you will not need liquids to assist in swallowing the food. For many people, eating and drinking together is a habit, not a necessity.

Describe your most negative experience with GBS.

Quote from Margaret B.:
    "The constant nausea for the first eight weeks and the despair over trying new meds, food, fluids, and a return to the hospital after three weeks. Eventually after many drugs and time it [the nausea] mostly passed and I felt human and 'lighter' and ready for the work ahead — lost weight but had a gain in self-understanding simultaneously."

4

Eating After
Gastric Bypass

Be aware that, for the rest of your life, protein must be given priority when choosing foods. The *minimum* protein requirement for men is 63 grams each day; for women, it is 50 grams. This amount is required to build and maintain muscle mass and to help maintain your weight after you have reached your goal. Be warned: It is usually not possible to consume that much protein from foods alone during the first month. The majority of patients use a protein supplement of some sort during the first few months. It is not a good idea to become too dependent on getting protein from these supplements, though, since the goal is to eat regular, healthful foods in appropriate amounts. It is better to choose nutritious foods from the start and to get used to eating them early in the process. Since the quantity consumed is so small, foods should be well-chosen and of good quality.

Good protein sources include:
- Poultry: chicken and turkey (skin is not allowed)
- Meats: beef, pork, lamb, veal, ham, low-fat sausages

- Fish: all kinds, including shellfish, and canned tuna and salmon (without bones)
- Peanut butter: creamy only, in small quantities
- Eggs: cooked any style
- Cheese, cottage cheese, yogurt: preferably low-fat or fat-free
- Milk: low-fat or fat-free
- Beans: all varieties of dried, including black, kidney, cannelloni, pinto, split peas, and fat-free refried beans
- Soy products: tofu, soy milk, soy yogurt, soy cheese

In general:
- 1 ounce meat, poultry, fish = approximately 7 grams of protein
- 1 egg = 7 grams of protein
- 2 tablespoons peanut butter = 7 grams of protein
- 1/4 cup low-fat cottage cheese = 6.5 grams of protein
- 1 ounce milk = 1 gram of protein

For many foods, the label will indicate grams of protein per serving. Pay attention to the portion size listed on the package, as compared to the amount you consume, when calculating your protein intake. Additionally, there are numerous books that list the protein content of thousands of foods. These are helpful for foods that are not required by law to be labeled, such as poultry, fish, and meats. Protein counter books can also help to calculate the protein content of some homemade foods, such as stew, which may not be made with a specific recipe. Check the listing in the protein book for canned beef stews, note the portion size given, and roughly estimate from the products listed the protein content of your homemade item. The same estimation can be made with soups and foods like chili and casseroles. The book can at least give you an approximate number without too much calculation. Additionally, many cookbooks provide a nutritional analysis of the recipes. That information is accurate to determine protein content.

The texture required of "puréed" foods can be compared to that of applesauce. Depending on the food itself, simply puréeing it in a food processor or blender can make the food sticky or paste-like. That texture is not acceptable. It may be necessary to add liquid in the form of broth, juice, milk, or even water to get the purée thin enough so that it will pass through the stomach easily. It is not necessary to invest in a large food processor. A good blender or small/mini food processor will be adequate to meet your needs for the first few weeks.

The following foods are acceptable in texture for the first two weeks:
- Applesauce
- Oatmeal, cream of wheat, grits
- Soups that contain no chunks — chunky soups will have to be put in the blender
- Instant mashed potatoes (can be made in small amounts conveniently)
- Canned, water-packed, chunk light tuna and canned chicken (can be made into moist salad with light mayo)
- Scrambled eggs
- Sugar-free Jello — provides little nutrition, but is generally acceptable

- Saltine or oyster crackers — only these types allowed in first two weeks
- Low-fat, low-sugar dairy yogurt (not frozen yogurt)
- Tofu and other smooth soy products

Commercial baby foods can be a convenient alternative. However, after gastric bypass, some people may find their taste and texture unappealing.

The following foods ARE NOT ACCEPTABLE:
- Raw fruits and vegetables of any kind unless blenderized, as in a shake
- Soft bread or rolls
- Pasta, rice, or noodles unless in soups — even in soups, they may be hard to digest unless they are very soft
- Fatty protein sources like hot dogs, sausage, and scrapple
- Regular milk shakes
- Raw eggs added to shakes to increase protein
- Carbonated drinks, full-strength fruit juices, sugar-sweetened drinks

FOODS CUT INTO SMALL PIECES ARE NOT CONSIDERED PURÉED.

If eating puréed foods does not appeal to you, rely on things like eggs, cheese, cottage cheese, moist tuna and chicken salad, soups, and other soft foods that do not have to be put into the blender. As you learn how and what to eat, it is important to make the eating experience a pleasant one. If your appetite is poor and/or you are finding this type of food unappealing, contact your dietitian for suggestions or ideas to make it more palatable. It is not advisable to drink just liquids and avoid food altogether. You must eventually learn what works for you and what doesn't. It is important to be patient with the process and with yourself.

The following tips will help you adjust to your new way of eating and drinking. Paying attention to them and making the changes permanent will contribute to your success with adapting to a new way of eating.

- Have a beverage with you at all times to sip on; do not gulp liquids.
- Do not use a drinking straw because it may cause belching.
- Do not eat and drink at the same time. Give yourself 20 to 30 minutes before and after eating to either stop or resume drinking.
- Chew foods slowly and thoroughly.
- Saltine crackers and thin-sliced, toasted bread are better accepted than soft bread.
- There are no foods that are uniformly not tolerated; some people can eat foods that others cannot.
- Eating more frequently helps most people adjust to the changes in eating.
- You may have to remind yourself to eat, since your appetite will be changing.
- Dilute fruit juices with water to increase fluid intake.
- Do not drink carbonated beverages or sugar-sweetened drinks. The carbonation may stretch the pouch and the sweet drinks provide no nutrition.

- If you feel full, stop eating; finishing even a small amount of food may make you feel uncomfortable.
- Use smaller plates to cut down on portion sizes.
- Use kid-sized forks and spoons, which slows the pace of eating and forces you to take smaller mouthfuls.
- Do not eat when watching television or reading, which may distract you from chewing properly and/or cause you to eat too fast or too much.
- Try changing the temperature of your beverages if you are not consuming enough fluids.
- Some people feel better if the first liquid they drink in the morning is warm, or room temperature, instead of ice-cold.
- It is not unusual for your sense of taste and smell to be heightened and for certain smells and tastes to be repulsive.

This is a common time to get frustrated and feel overwhelmed. Again, the support of family and friends is critical. Attending a support group for gastric bypass patients during this period can be very helpful, as well. Do not wait until you feel you are recovered from the surgery to go to a meeting. This period of time may be the hardest to get through, and you may find it very beneficial to talk to someone who has had similar experiences.

5

Vitamin, Mineral, and Protein Supplementation

It will be necessary to take a good quality multiple vitamin and mineral product for the rest of your life, and to take additional calcium and Vitamin B-12 supplements. The reduced food intake of a gastric bypass patient makes it impossible to get adequate amounts of vitamins and minerals from diet alone. This matter cannot be negotiated. Vitamin deficiencies can result in serious medical implications. Some deficiencies are noticed more quickly than others, while some may take a while to be detected.

Additionally, for the first few months, you may need to augment your protein intake with a protein supplement product. Don't rely on these products for too long, however. As your diet standardizes, it is advisable to wean yourself off of them and begin to eat more regular foods. A balanced, well-chosen diet should be able to supply you with adequate amounts of protein. However, the supplements can be helpful to use when your schedule is disrupted, when meals will be missed, when traveling, or when protein-rich foods may not be available. Most people find it convenient to have a liquid supplement or a protein bar handy for those situations.

Vitamin and Mineral Supplements

Vitamins are nutrients which contribute to good health by regulating the metabolism and assisting with the release of energy from digested food. The body needs them in relatively small amounts, as compared to nutrients such as protein, carbohydrates, and fat. Vitamins are either water-soluble or fat-soluble. Water-soluble vitamins cannot be stored by the body and must be taken daily. They include the B vitamins and vitamin C. Fat-soluble vitamins are stored in the body's fatty tissue and include vitamins A, D, E, and K. All vitamins need to be taken regularly.

Minerals are needed for the proper composition of body fluids, the formation of blood and bone, the regulation of muscle tone (including that of the cardiovascular system), and the maintenance of healthy nerve function. Minerals are essential for efficient utilization by the body of vitamins and other nutrients. Proper equilibrium of the body's systems depends on the levels of different minerals and the ratios of certain mineral levels to one another. The level of each mineral in the body has an effect on every other, so if one mineral is out of balance, all can be affected.

With food intake severely restricted, it is mandatory to take good quality vitamin and mineral supplements for the rest of your life. At first, a chewable form is recommended, since it will be better tolerated and absorbed. It is not necessary, however, to take a chewable preparation forever. If you prefer it, as many people do, it is certainly acceptable. Others change to a swallow vitamin and mineral tablet after about six to nine months. Ask your dietitian to recommend a good product. It is not acceptable to use a product designed for children, since the amounts of vitamins and minerals are not adequate for adults. The multivitamin and mineral product should provide at least the minimum recommended Daily Values set by the FDA.

Vitamin B-12

Vitamin B-12 absorption is significantly impaired after Roux-en-Y gastric bypass, for a number of reasons. Intake of foods that are good sources of B-12, such as red meats, is limited. There is a less acidic environment in the pouch, as compared to the normal stomach, which makes it more difficult to absorb the vitamin. *Intrinsic factor* is a protein produced in the gastrointestinal tract that is necessary for B-12 absorption, as well. The portion of the tract that produces this factor is bypassed by Roux-en-Y, so taking a swallow form of the vitamin is not acceptable.

Regular injections or sublingual (under the tongue) tablets are the preferred methods for supplementation. The sublingual tablets are available in over-the-counter doses of 500 micrograms (mcg). They are designed to dissolve quickly and will be absorbed by the soft tissue in the mouth. They should not be chewed. The tablets are to be taken daily; the injections are given monthly. Many individuals find they are able to give themselves the injections.

Vitamin B-12 is needed to prevent anemia. It aids in regulating the formation of red blood cells and helps in the utilization of iron. It is also needed for proper digestion; the absorption of foods; the metabolism of protein, carbohydrates, and fats; and maintenance of the nervous system. Common symptoms of a B-12 deficiency are an unsteady gait and a tingling sensation in the feet or legs.

Calcium

Calcium deficiency is common and can be prevented by consuming the correct form and amount of calcium. Calcium citrate is the best supplement form, since it does not require acid to break it down. Many supplements contain calcium carbonate, which is not as effective. It is necessary to take 1,200 to 1,500 milligrams of calcium daily, in divided doses, because the body will not absorb more than 500 to 600 milligrams at a time. Taking the supplements at regular times of the day, such as at breakfast, lunch, and dinner, can assist you in remembering to take them.

Chewable forms of calcium are recommended at first. They are available over-the-counter in 500 to 600 milligram tablets.

Iron

Not all patients need supplemental iron. It is usually prescribed on an individual basis. Some patients have difficulty tolerating iron supplements, experiencing constipation from them, in particular. If an iron supplement is indicated and side effects are experienced, it is important to inform your doctor so that a stool softener or another form of iron can be recommended.

Iron and calcium compete with each other for absorption by the body. Take these supplements two to three hours apart.

Biotin

Temporary hair loss can be experienced after GBS. It may happen for several reasons. First, it may be related to the anesthesia from the surgery (people who have other types of surgery also sometimes experience hair loss). It can also be related to vitamin and protein intake. Biotin is a vitamin that is needed for healthy hair and skin. A daily supplement of 100 milligrams of biotin may prevent hair loss. It is available over-the-counter in the form of tablets to be swallowed.

If you stop taking the vitamin and mineral supplements for any reason, be sure to notify your doctor so that any problems can be corrected. If your doctor did not emphasize taking vitamins, ask your dietitian to recommend a good product. Your vitamin and mineral intake will affect your nutritional status for the rest of your life. Ignoring that fact, or feeling that it is not important to take supplements regularly, is a mistake you can't afford to make.

Protein Supplements

For the first few months after surgery, until you have completely healed and your eating patterns have stabilized, you will most likely need to take a protein supplement. There are many products available to supplement protein intake. Select one that provides at least 15 grams of protein per serving and is low in carbohydrates. (If the supplement is labeled as *low carb*, it is acceptable.)

Read the label carefully. Some of the powders must be mixed with 8 to 12 ounces of liquid, which may be too much to drink at one time. Saving some of it for later use may not be a good idea, however, since many of the supplements thicken on standing and become unpalatable. New products are continuously being developed, and you should be able to find a supplement that meets your particular needs. Check with your dietitian before using a particular supplement. There may be unacceptable ingredients in the product or it may not meet the requirements of your surgeon.

It is good to be prepared with a supplement of some sort to use immediately after you are discharged from the hospital. However, be aware that your tastes may change from day to day and week to week. It is not wise to buy any protein supplement, or food item, for that matter, in large quantities. A supplement you tasted and found acceptable before surgery may seem unappealing afterwards. Note that products purchased on the Internet may be difficult or impossible to return. It is most beneficial to purchase products locally. Your dietitian can advise you about local sources for acceptable products; additionally, some surgeons sell the products they want their patients to use.

What advice would you have to offer to individuals considering the surgery?

Quote from Ann G.:

"It is not a gift. It's a key. You still have to follow every rule and really work at it. It's a lifelong commitment to a changed lifestyle. Your thoughts will still be obese. You will have to learn to think thin."

6

Two-Week
Follow-Up Visit

Describe your most positive experience with GBS.

Quote from Kathy L.:

"Losing weight — the ease of not being hungry. Eating a healthy diet without fear of gaining weight. I can even have snacks within reason without fear of it going to my hips."

Patients are usually required to see the surgeon two weeks after surgery. At that time, they may be given permission to drive a vehicle and resume regular activities. Moderate exercise is recommended at this point. Heavy lifting is not allowed for a while longer. The process of recuperation and transition to the new way of eating is dynamic and can be expected to change from day to day. Most people feel well physically at this point, although they may be a little tired and still sore from the surgical procedure itself. It is also very common for them to feel blue, depressed, emotional, or confused. It's a good idea to keep notes during the first two weeks, so you will remember what questions and concerns to bring up with your surgeon and other support people. Patients generally look forward to this appointment because they have had the chance to eat, drink, and try out new foods; perhaps have experienced some difficulties; wish to report early successes; and are eager to pass on tips about what has and has not worked for them.

Some patients feel wonderful after two weeks and are ready to get back to a normal routine. Try not to be overconfident at this point and try to do too much, too soon. It is still very important to follow the directions of your professional support team. Expect them to give you guidelines and recommendations to follow. If they do not, ask for them.

At this point, you will begin to reintroduce foods into your diet one at a time. This is done so that, if you have a problem with a particular food, it will be easy to identify. If you eat two new foods at the same time, you may not know which one caused the problem. Take, for example, tomato sauce and lean ground beef. If you have already tolerated tomato sauce, it's fine to have the sauce and beef together. If you haven't, and you find you don't feel well after eating the sauce and ground beef, you will not be sure if it was the beef or the sauce that didn't agree with you.

After the two-week follow-up appointment, you will also begin to try foods that are cut in small pieces, rather than puréed/blenderized. It's best to begin with foods you tolerated well in the puréed form. For example, if you could eat puréed chicken, try some in small pieces. For those who have not had any blenderized poultry or meats, try poultry and fish before beef and pork, as they are generally easier to digest. Remember that everyone's reaction to a particular food is different and you need to be patient with the process of trying new foods. Now and in the future, remember that the more moist the food is, the easier it will be to tolerate.

Dumping Syndrome

The "Dumping Syndrome" can occur after gastric bypass surgery. Foods that are high in sugar are usually not well-tolerated. Dumping is characterized by a set of symptoms, including a shaky, sweaty, dizzy sensation accompanied by a rapid heart rate and, oftentimes, severe diarrhea. When sugar is consumed, it passes, or is "dumped," rapidly into the small intestine, causing an overload, which results in a fluid shift from the blood into the intestine. The decrease in blood volume increases the heart rate, resulting in the individual feeling strongly like she needs to lie down (which would improve cardiac output). The influx of fluid into the intestine due to the sugar overload can lead to a watery diarrhea. To compound the problem, the insulin response to large amounts of sugar entering the bloodstream causes symptoms of hypoglycemia, leaving the individual feeling faint and weak.

Dumping Syndrome is of benefit, since it provides negative feedback to eating sugar. Those who experience it want to avoid another episode, so they quickly learn to avoid sugar. Sensitivity to sugar can vary. There are some who never experience any problems.

Some people try foods that are labeled "sugar-free" to indulge their desire for sweets. These foods can contain sugar alcohols, which, even in small amounts, can cause diarrhea in anyone, whether they have had gastric bypass or not. Look for the words sorbitol, mannitol, and maltitol on labels and stay away from those products.

Sucralose is not a sugar alcohol. It is a reconfigured sugar molecule which is safe to use. It should not cause diarrhea and can be used to make sugar-free foods. You can even bake with it. The molecule is not metabolized like sugar and will not cause Dumping Syndrome. It is sold under the brand name *Splenda*.

Two-Week Follow-Up Nutrition Reminders:

1. Continue to drink plenty of water and noncarbonated, sugar-free fluids. The fluids can be hot, warm, or cold, whichever suits you best. Your eventual goal is to consume 64 ounces per day of non-caffeinated fluids.

2. Continue to use a protein shake. If you begin eating more protein-rich foods in the coming weeks, you may not need the shake every day. It is a good idea to continue to have it regularly until you are consuming adequate protein from food sources.

3. Do not forget that, although you are not hungry, it is important to eat at regular intervals. Your food intake can influence the rate at which you lose weight. Undereating can be as much of a problem as overeating. The key is to achieve the proper balance of calories taken in to calories being used.

4. If you are returning to work soon, try your best to have a food/meal schedule worked out. Returning to work too soon

may present a problem if you cannot eat at regular intervals, or if you do not have appropriate foods available when you are away from home. Plan ahead and try to mimic a workday schedule while you are still at home.

5. If you are reluctant to try different foods, you may find yourself getting bored with what you are eating. At home, try a small amount of something new every so often. If you tolerate the food well, add it to your diet. If it does not agree with you, avoid it for a few weeks and then try it again. Your food preferences will continue to change over time.

6. Fried foods and foods that are high in fat (regular sausage, hot dogs, scrapple) should not be eaten. There are better protein choices than those foods. The high fat content of these and other foods is often the reason some people feel sick after eating. When eating in a restaurant, foods may be prepared with more fat or oil than you are used to when eating at home. Ask questions about preparation methods of the food when you are ordering from a restaurant menu. If you do not want to elaborate on your reason for asking questions about food content, just say that you are allergic to certain ingredients and you have to avoid them.

7. You can try different protein bars as a convenient food to carry with you. Again, don't buy any one kind in large quantities, as you may lose your taste for it after a while. Protein bars vary greatly in taste and content. Try to find one that provides at least 15 grams of protein and has around

200 calories. It is not unusual to only eat part of a bar at a time. Some of the bars can be dry and hard to digest, so you may need to try different kinds.

8. Sugar-free candy can cause diarrhea, even in small amounts. Hard candy sweetened with sucralose is usually well-tolerated. If you find you have a bad taste in your mouth or your breath is bad, you may have a sugar-free mint. Some people use the paper-like, mint-flavored breath strips.

9. Avoid the following foods: sweets, full-strength fruit juices of any kind (only diluted juices are allowed to avoid Dumping Syndrome), fatty cuts of meat, fried foods, hot dogs, scrapple, regular mayonnaise or salad dressing (use the light versions).

10. It is *extremely important* to keep a food record, particularly if you are having digestive problems of any kind. This is the most accurate tool for tracking and solving problems related to food intake. It is a good idea to take a three-day food diary to every doctor's appointment, not just the two-week follow-up appointment. Remember that the nutrition component of your diet will be of increased importance for the rest of your life. Having the dietitian check your intake in the months after the surgery may prevent future problems.

11. Remember to be patient with your transition to the new way of eating after GBS. It is a process which changes constantly. Try not to get discouraged when you are having difficulties.

If you experience symptoms of depression or find yourself getting emotional, know that this is a very normal reaction to the procedure. Ask for support or professional help if the problems or negative thoughts persist.

12. If you experience vomiting, do not go right back to solid foods when you feel like eating again. Slowly begin to drink and eat, using broths, tea, and unsweetened fluids that appeal to you. Drink and eat slowly; do not let yourself get dehydrated. Try small amounts of food at first, like saltines, oatmeal or cream of wheat, toasted bread, or applesauce. Avoid dairy products for a few days because they may not agree with you after a bout of vomiting.

13. If you experience diarrhea, avoid milk products for a few days when you reintroduce foods. Remember to stay away from fatty foods, as well. Follow the guidelines in #12 to prevent dehydration.

From this point on, it is critical to the success of the GBS patient that food consumed be of high quality. It is disturbing to read a food record of someone who is one month out from the procedure who is eating snack foods, fast food, and ignoring the protein content of his or her diet. Eventually, these poor choices will catch up with that person. Hair loss, lack of energy, dry skin, and fatigue are common complaints of those who are not mindful of the content of their diets. As you are adjusting to this different way of eating, it is important to get accustomed to good quality food.

Initially, patients take longer to eat. It may take some people up to 40 minutes to consume just a small amount of food. Eventually, it will take less time. At first, some people say, "I feel as though I am always eating." That is common; however, after the first few weeks, meals should only last for 20 to 25 minutes. If you take longer, it may be that you are eating too much or not listening to your cues for fullness.

Grazing behavior, which can mean always munching on something, or eating a small amount of food, waiting 10 minutes, and going back for another bite, is highly discouraged. It can lead to stretching of the pouch, eventually enabling you to consume larger amounts of food than you should. Grazing is a behavior that should be stopped as soon as it is recognized. In the case of some people who regain weight after GBS, it is because this behavior was either ignored or not recognized. For those who are "stress eaters," it is critical to learn another method to deal with stress.

What has been the greatest benefit you have experienced after having GBS?

Quote from Donna B:
   "To still be able to eat what I want, just in moderation. Other diets never worked because they restrict certain foods. I almost resented that and would eat it anyway because I felt deprived. I feel more in control now."

7

Making Lifestyle Changes More Permanent

After the first few months, everything will seem easier. You will feel more energetic and be more confident in your food choices. You will be taking fewer prescription drugs. Your clothes will be much looser. And, you will feel sure that you made the right decision to have gastric bypass.

However, it is at this point that you have to continue to work at making lifestyle changes permanent. The scheduling of follow-up appointments depends upon the surgeon. Some require more visits than others. If your surgeon does not have a specific routine for follow-up, and you feel that you need it, ask for help. There are online support groups and support group meetings at local hospitals that are usually open to anyone. Talk to others who have had the surgery and get references for professionals who can help with your problem areas. If you need mental health or nutrition advice, try to find professionals who have experience with gastric bypass.

Please include any additional comments.

Quote from Ryan G:

"In all the experiences I mentioned, I left out the most important part. The new friends I have made. This would not have been as easy as it was with a different staff at the office and hospital. Drs. Singh and Averbach, Cathy, Brandy, and Carol, and you made this so much easier. Your willingness to listen to any and all questions at any point in time was so meaningful that words can't really describe it. Also meeting people at the support group meetings has given me more motivation. I want to do even better so I can tell them when I see them."

Not all dietitians and nutritionists are familiar with the nutritional needs of the gastric bypass patient. Gastric bypass is not traditional stomach surgery for gastrointestinal problems. (Dietary requirements for each are very different.) Diabetics who have had gastric bypass cannot follow a typical diabetic diet after the surgery because it would mean eating too much food and in the wrong proportions of protein, carbohydrate, and fat. It is not a traditional method for weight loss, either. Eating after GBS must include adequate protein first and may not include the variety and amount of foods on a typical diet plan. Emphasis on food tolerance and preference after GBS is important. I have had patients referred to me who had been given completely erroneous advice from dietitians who had no idea about nutritional requirements or restrictions after gastric bypass.

Exercise

Developing an acceptable routine for regular exercise is very important. Most people who are morbidly obese have not been able to exercise with any regularity. Being able to exercise and move freely, without pain, is one of the reasons people choose to have gastric bypass.

However, there are still many people who, after the surgery, are afraid to exercise and resist or make excuses. Those who are most successful with gastric bypass are those who incorporate exercise into their lives early in the recuperation stage. The activity you choose is up to you. It should be something you enjoy and do not dread doing. The activity can change, and probably will, as your body becomes smaller and your stamina and energy improve. If you are not sure what exercise to do, or have questions or concerns about your physical capabilities, it may be to your advantage to contact a certified personal trainer to design an appropriate exercise program that meets your specific needs. Working with a personal trainer does not require a long-term commitment and may be well worth the cost to provide you with an appropriate, comfortable, yet challenging exercise routine. Some patients are thrilled to be able to go to a gym and work out. For much of their lives, going to a gym and appearing in public to exercise was unthinkable. Many of those who have had the surgery are impressed with their ability to increase their level of exercise within a short period of time and to fit in with other members at the gym.

It is not uncommon at this point for people to say, "I didn't think I would have to work so hard at this. Surgery was not the easy way out." Now is the time to remember that gastric bypass surgery is a tool. The procedure enables you to lose weight and keep it off and takes you to the point where proper diet and exercise *do* work. Diet and exercise may not have worked for you in the past; now, that combination is what it will take for you to be successful. It can be discouraging for some to feel that they have to work so hard at losing weight and keeping it off. You may have to remind yourself that you knew from the start that gastric bypass was not a "quick fix" and that the improvement in your health and well-being is worth all the effort.

This is not the time to get complacent or to return to some of your old habits. It is critical to notice and admit when old behaviors are returning and to realize that you need to regroup and make changes. This is the time to ask for help from the professionals on your team and to admit that you need some reinforcement and encouragement. It is not unusual for this to happen. It is not a sign of failure. Rather, you should feel good that you have noticed and taken steps to prevent slowing your progress or backsliding. If you are not exercising regularly, find that your food choices are not as good as they should be, are giving in to others who may be sabotaging your efforts, or are accepting some weight loss as good enough, it is time to ask for support and guidance.

Cosmetic Surgery

It is a common concern of many people that losing a great deal of weight will result in excessive amounts of loose, drooping skin. Do not assume that plastic or reconstructive surgery will be necessary. The amount of excess skin is determined by several factors. They include: the length of time you were overweight, how overweight you were prior to the surgery, the type of skin you have genetically, how much exercise you get, and the content of your diet.

Cosmetic surgery should not be considered for a minimum of 18 months after gastric bypass. At that point, the body has adjusted to its lower weight and, typically, weight loss has slowed or stopped. Cosmetic surgery performed too soon after gastric bypass could have disappointing results. The body needs a chance to stabilize and, if you are still getting regular exercise, your body shape may continue to change. Muscle toning can make clothes fit differently, even though you may not be losing pounds.

Insurance coverage for cosmetic surgery after weight loss varies. For those who have a large amount of excess tissue in the stomach area, it is important to be aware of tissue breakdown and the risk of serious infection. Viewing that area on the body may be difficult; however, it is critical to your overall health to closely observe any changes in your skin. If there are areas that seem to be chafing or breaking down, inform your doctor and have it noted in your medical record. The fact that there is an increased risk of infection when the skin is not in good condition may improve the chances for insurance coverage for cosmetic surgery.

Whole body lifts, chin reconstruction, breast reduction, and facelifts are procedures commonly requested by patients who have lost significant amounts of weight. As with any surgery, you owe it to yourself to do as much research as you can to select the proper procedure and find the most qualified surgeon.

Personal references are the best way to find a good plastic surgeon. Interview several before you make a final decision and discuss in detail what you expect from the reconstructive surgery.

8

Emotional & Psychological Aspects of Eating Differently

Food has so much meaning in today's world. Most, if not all, gastric bypass patients have used food for many reasons other than hunger. We eat because we are:

- Happy
- Sad
- Angry
- Frustrated
- Lonely
- Depressed
- Anxious
- Stressed

The key after GBS is to learn how to deal with these emotions when you can no longer use food to suppress them.

I have been told countless times, "I didn't know how much my life revolved around food until I had this surgery." This is another factor you must take into account when considering GBS. Eating out and socializing will be affected by the surgery.

I have many patients who are gourmet cooks who were very concerned about the fact that they spent so much time around food. In the end, it works out fine. They learn how to eat differently, cook more creatively, and still enjoy the art of cooking, but eat smaller amounts of the good quality food they prepare. The pleasure they get out of feeling healthier and having more energy usually makes up for the reduced amount of food they can eat.

The spouses of many patients sometimes express concern about not being able to eat out as much, or at all. This is a common worry among patients who do not cook and rely on restaurant food and/or convenience foods. A nutritionist can help these people make better choices and educate them about getting the most nutrition from small amounts of food. Many times this does not present the problem that they thought it would. It is not unusual for a patient to say, "I can't believe I am actually craving salads now. I never used to eat vegetables." GBS patients feel better when they eat better and make good food choices. One patient who ate lots of beef before the surgery told me he was amazed that he orders salads with chicken now because that is what he wants to eat, regardless of other foods on the menu.

What advice would you give to individuals considering the surgery?

Quote from Karen J.:
"Make sure you are mentally prepared and have sought some sort of counseling for your eating disorder — YOU DO HAVE ONE. Learn new coping mechanisms that don't include food."

Describe your most negative experience with GBS.

Quote from Bambi W.:

"Immediate depression and anxiety! What did I do to my body! Nothing you read can prepare you if this happens. I was actually grieving. I lost a best friend — FOOD."

Additional comments or observations you would like to make concerning GBS.

Quote from Cheryl W.:

"I don't think this surgery is for everyone!! You need to be ready (mentally) for the changes that take place. You can't rely on your old habits to deal with your life challenges. I hated the fact that I couldn't control my eating — now it's not in my control and I love it!! I can still eat whatever I want (within reason) but not a whole lot! My husband says I am a cheap date."

Quote from Kelly A.:

"I don't regret having the surgery. I do believe that as you continue to lose weight, depending on how long you've been overweight, some therapy is needed as you adjust your body image. The surgery can and will give you your life back. I encourage and applaud all those who are contemplating or have gotten the surgery done."

P.O.W.E.R.

Throughout the first year after GBS, the changes and challenges are continuous. The process of adapting to a whole new way of life evokes every possible emotion. It is helpful to have reinforcement and reassurance that the surgery was the right choice.

I have developed an acronym which can serve as a reminder that you are doing everything possible to be successful. I chose the word "POWER" because you are now exercising more power over every aspect of your life than you ever have before. Repeating the acronym as positive reinforcement can help you to succeed.

Protein

Protein is the most important nutrient to consume on a daily basis to maintain muscle mass and promote healing. Muscle tissue is more metabolically active than fat tissue, so as body fat decreases, your metabolism changes for the better. Protein foods will contribute most of your calories for the rest of your life. Women require a minimum of 50 grams per day; men, a minimum of 63 grams. Even more protein can be safely consumed, if you are able. Protein sources include meat, poultry, fish, cheese, eggs, peanut butter, beans, tofu and other soy products, and milk. The choices may become boring, but the majority of people feel better when they consume adequate protein. Protein drinks and bars are concentrated sources of protein which can be used if intake of regular foods is limited.

When you return home immediately after the surgery, it is a good idea to have a protein drink available to use daily. Down the road, the protein drinks and bars can always be used if you are not getting enough protein from food sources. It is not recommended to rely on the bars and drinks as your primary protein sources, however. Eating regular, good quality food should be the long-term goal.

Ownership

Choosing to have gastric bypass surgery is a decision made by the individual, for the individual, to enhance that person's life and improve his health. Therefore, the individual must take full responsibility for making changes and choices. People undergoing GBS must accept that the decision is about their own bodies. The surgery is changing their bodies for the better. It is critical to have the support and encouragement of others, but, ultimately, it is the individual who will make the choices about food, exercise, and attitude. No one should make food choices for you. No one can exercise for you. No one can change your attitude for you. Prior to the surgery, it will be helpful to inform your family and those close to you that things will be changing, if everyone has relied on you to do things for them. It is now time for you to take care of yourself.

What advice would you have to offer to family members of those who have had GBS?

Quote from Patricia A.:
   "My family was totally against the surgery. They were afraid I

was going to die. What they didn't realize and what I told them is that I would rather be dead than to live what remains of my life trapped in my obese body. I was willing to risk everything for the chance to get my life back. So my advice for family members is to do your own research. Find out first-hand what the surgery entails, what the risks are, etc. And LISTEN to the one who is contemplating the surgery. Really listen. Be supportive. And after the surgery, do not become the food police. No one knows better than the person having the surgery what they can and cannot or should and should not eat."

What advice would you have to offer to individuals considering the surgery?

Quote from Lisa V.:

"Do it for yourself! Consider all of your options. Realize that this is only a tool. It won't work forever, you have to do your part to make it successful. Be good to yourself, make sure you have a way to deal with stress, because if you are a 'stress eater' you'll have to find another option."

Water

Water is a nutrient and is essential for proper body function. It helps to eliminate waste, remove toxins, lubricate joints, and moisturize the skin. The daily recommendation for water intake is 64 ounces. Having water with you at all times is a requirement.

Keep in mind, though, that eating and drinking at the same time is discouraged. It is necessary for each person to decide for himself the best method to use to consume adequate amounts of water on a daily basis. Some prefer ice water; others prefer water to be warm or room temperature. Inadequate water intake can slow weight loss and contribute to constipation, dry skin, and frequent colds. If you are having difficulty consuming enough water, ask your dietitian for suggestions to improve your intake.

Exercise

Exercise is critical to success with GBS. Aerobic exercise is needed to burn calories, and weight-bearing exercise is needed to build and maintain muscle mass. The endorphins that are released during exercise contribute to well-being and positive attitude. Most people who are morbidly obese have not been able to exercise with any regularity. It is highly encouraged to engage in some sort of physical activity from the start to improve flexibility and boost metabolism. Many people who have had the surgery are impressed with their ability to increase their level of exercise within a short period of time. Many often get so accustomed to the positive effects of regular exercise that they feel poorly when they miss even a few days of it.

What has been the greatest benefit you have experienced after having GBS?

Quote from Dyanna M.:
"The greatest benefit for me has been regaining the active life

I had before I became obese. I am able to run, jog, swim, bike, and perform many more physical activities that had become so difficult for me as my weight increased over the years. I am living and breathing like someone with a zest for life once again!"

Quote from Deborah L.:

"Physically, I feel great. I don't get out of breath or tired. I am much more active. Emotionally, I am on cloud nine."

Results

Results will be achieved if you follow these recommendations:

Adequate **PROTEIN** intake + **OWNERSHIP** of your decision + sufficient **WATER** intake + regular **EXERCISE** = **RESULTS**

Include any additional comments or observations you would like to make.

Quote from Christine F.:

"It was the best decision I have ever made. My value of life has improved immensely and continues to improve more and more each day. You are surprised at how many little things you can do that you could not have even attempted before."

Quote from Louise S.:

"My daughter thinks I'm 'cute.' We are now able to share clothes. Everyone thinks I look great. They now say, 'I'm so tiny and petite.'"

———————

Quote from Ann G.:

"The same granddaughter who said, 'Granny, I like you just the way you are,' when I was wearing size 22W, said with delight when I reached a size 8 petite in just four months, 'Granny, you've really changed. You're wearing earrings and lipstick and you've even changed radio stations!'"

9

There Is Life After Gastric Bypass Surgery

Bariatric surgery will continue to be used by the morbidly obese as a means to lose weight and improve health. It is a decision to be made with as much insight, information, and perspective as possible. The most fundamental skill we practice as humans — eating — has to be relearned. The surgery can have a remarkable and profound impact on the quality of life, but only if the individual is capable of making permanent lifestyle changes.

Gastric bypass is not for everyone. It is a life-altering procedure that should be considered the final resort and not something that can be tried out or reversed if you do not like it. If there is any doubt whatsoever that it may not be the right choice for you, do not have the surgery. The vast majority of people who have had the surgery are very happy with their decision. There are some, however, who are not. If you have psychological issues that are strongly connected to food, they should be resolved before having the surgery. After gastric bypass, food takes on a totally different meaning.

Dealing with the transition to a new way of life after gastric bypass can be very stressful. As time passes, new issues related to body image, self-acceptance, and relationships will develop. Counseling or therapy may be necessary to help resolve them. Do not underestimate the value of therapy to help overcome difficulties and contribute to your success.

There is life after gastric bypass surgery. The quality of that life is up to the individual. The choices and changes you make will be reflected in your success and happiness.

Appendix:
Frequently
Asked Questions

What should I do to prevent boredom from eating the same foods?

Many people complain of boredom with eating after gastric bypass surgery. Giving priority to protein-rich foods is important; however, it can be monotonous. A good way to add variety to your meals is with vegetables and fruits which are low in calories and packed with vitamins and minerals. Cooked vegetables and canned fruits are better choices at first, progressing to salads and fresh fruits slowly and in small amounts to establish your individual tolerance levels.

Is it normal to feel queasy in the morning?

Timing of meals and snacks cannot be overlooked when adjusting to eating after gastric bypass. Appetite changes and the concerns people have about late-night eating can mean going from early evening to the next morning without food. A light snack 1 or 1-1/2 hours before bedtime can be beneficial. It may prevent low blood sugar symptoms and the "empty" feeling one can experience upon waking in the morning. Suggestions for snacks include: crackers and low-fat cheese or peanut butter, low-fat cottage cheese (with or without fruit), a small bowl of cereal (can help with constipation problems), a protein shake or part of a protein bar. For some individuals, drinking a warm beverage first thing in the morning is helpful, rather than a cold drink.

Will I ever be able to drink a carbonated beverage again?

It is not a good idea to drink carbonated beverages, as this can stretch the pouch. If you are queasy and have settled your stomach in the past with cola or ginger ale, you may have it stirred (flat); it must be diet. Learning how to drink sodas after gastric bypass is not something to feel good about. In the long run, it will harm you.

Is having bad breath and/or a funny taste in the mouth common?

It is very common to have bad breath when you are losing weight quickly. It can be the result of ketones being given off as you burn fat. It can also be the result of being dehydrated or from having acid in your stomach. It is important to consume adequate fluids after gastric bypass and to always have a beverage — preferably water — to sip on with you at all times. It is critical immediately after surgery to not get dehydrated.

To alleviate the bad breath/taste, you can use breath strips or brush your teeth frequently with a soft toothbrush. Dentists recommend gently brushing your tongue, especially if you feel as though your mouth is very dry. A great deal of foul-smelling bacteria can accumulate on your tongue. It is important to pay attention to regular dental care, as well.

I find that I begin to sneeze when I feel full. Is that unusual?

Sneezing when you are full is not common; however, it is not unusual. Be grateful that your body is giving you a signal of this nature before you overeat and become uncomfortable.

Some people find that their nose runs when they eat. If this happens, it is not cause for concern, only an annoyance.

I am able to eat anything and that scares me.

Remember that gastric bypass is a tool. If you find that you are able to eat most foods, keep the amounts to a minimum and continue to listen to your body's cues for fullness. Months and years after the surgery, you should still be aware of the amounts and types of foods that you are eating and the time it takes you to eat. If you find that there is any area in which you need help, ask your dietitian for strategies to deal with the problem. It is not uncommon for this sort of issue to develop after gastric bypass.

Gastric bypass has provided you with a tool to make it easier for you to eat properly, lose weight, and keep it off. It is not a "quick fix." You will have to make good choices for the rest of your life. Paying attention to your food intake and exercise level over the long run will be critical to your success with the surgery.

Finding a comfort level with food and your ability to enjoy food and everything it means to you should be a goal. It is a powerful feeling to know that you are in control of your food choices and amounts. The food should no longer be controlling you, but, rather, you must control the food.

How do I overcome the "grazing" behavior?

Grazing over the course of the day is common. It is not a good idea in the long run. It can lead to overeating and never feeling satisfied.

After about the first six to eight weeks, it is best to take 20 to 25 minutes to eat a meal. The amount of food will be small. If you find that you take more than that time to eat, you may be overeating. It takes 20 minutes for the brain to get the signal that you are full. If you eat for longer than that, you may be forcing the food and, subsequently, eating more than you need.

Grazing is a common habit among people who are "oral" and always need something in their mouths. It is common, also, in settings where there is exposure to a lot of food on a regular basis throughout the day. If you find this happening to you, stop the behavior. Make an effort to eat for only 20 to 25 minutes. It is better to eat a small amount of food every three to four hours than to eat constantly and have a small amount of food in your pouch at all times. This is common behavior among those who are afraid to eat too much at one time and get overfull and uncomfortable. It is a behavior that should be recognized and dealt with. It can lead to overeating and regaining weight.

Can I get protein from a pill?

Proteins are composed of amino acids. They are available in pill form; however, pills do not provide complete proteins, nor are they utilized like proteins from food. Pills are prescribed for specific conditions and not for nourishment.

It is *not* possible to take a pill to nourish yourself. You must learn how to eat and drink properly to maintain muscle mass and prevent the development of future problems related to nutrition.

Prior to gastric bypass surgery, you were made aware that this is not the easy way to deal with weight loss. It is the ultimate challenge to eat properly when you have no appetite and to satisfy your nutritional requirements with small amounts of food. It is imperative that you ask for support and assistance if you feel that you are not consuming enough food, especially protein.

How can I increase my fluid intake? I know I am not drinking enough.

It may be that the temperature of the fluid is the problem. Some people can only drink fluids that are ice cold, and there are others who need room temperature or warm liquids. Remember that any caffeine-free fluid counts toward your eventual goal of 64 ounces per day. That includes protein drinks, soups, juicy fruits, Jello, sugar-free drinks, and diluted fruit juices. Whatever it takes, pay attention to your fluid intake. It is never good to get dehydrated.

What can I do to prevent hair loss?

The protein intake and multivitamin and mineral you are taking is critical. If you are not taking a good vitamin regularly, inform your doctor. It is of utmost importance, since you cannot make up for weeks or months of insufficient intake. The protein intake is important to prevent hair loss. Sometimes, dramatic, rapid weight loss can cause hair loss, along with the anesthesia and the stress of surgery. The advice to eat protein should not be taken lightly, since there are eventual consequences if intake is not adequate.

Biotin, a B-vitamin, taken regularly, may help with hair loss. It may not prevent hair loss completely. It is recommended for healthy hair, skin, and nails.

You may consult with your hair stylist for advice regarding specific products and techniques to prevent hair loss.

Suggested Resources

ADA Publications and Resources

ADA's Managing Obesity: A clinical guide. Available at http://www.eatright.org/Public/ProductCatalog/104_17783.cfm. Accessed June 20, 2004.

Dietetic Practice Group — The Weight Management: DPG prevention and treatment of overweight and obesity throughout the life cycle. Available at: http://www.eatright.org/Member/index_dpg26.cfm. Accessed June 20, 2004.

Marcason W. What Are the Dietary Guidelines Following Bariatric Surgery? *J Am Diet Assoc*. 2004;104:487–488.

Nutritional Implications of Bariatric Surgery: Perspectives of practitioners audiotape/handout. Available at: https://www.krm.com/regonline/amdvcregs.nsf/amd8014-0. Accessed June 20, 2004.

Weight Management — Position of ADA. *J Am Diet Assoc*. 2002;102:1145–1155. Available at: http://www.eatright.org/Public/GovernmentAffairs/92_adar0802.cfm. Accessed June 20, 2004.

Other Resources

Brolin RE, Gorman JH, Gorman RC, Petschenik AJ, Bradley LJ, Kenler HA, Cody RP. Are Vitamin B-12 and Folate Deficiency Clinically Important After Roux-en-Y Gastric Bypass? *J Gastrointest Surg*. 1998;2:436–442.

Elliott K. Nutritional Considerations After Bariatric Surgery. *Crit Care Nurs Q*. 2003;26:133–138.

Flegal KM, Carroll MD, Ogden CL, Johnson CL. Prevalence and Trends in Obesity Among U.S. Adults, 1999–2000. *JAMA*. 2002;288:1723–1727.

Stocker DJ. Management of the Bariatric Surgery Patient. *Endocrinol Metab Clin N Am*. 2003;32:437–457.

Bariatric Practice Guidelines. American Society of Bariatric Physicians. Available at: http://www.asbp.org/states/practiceguidelines.htm. Accessed June 20, 2004.

AGA Technical Review on Obesity. *Gastroenterology*. 2002;123:882–932.

Deitel M, Shikora SA. Review: The development of the surgical treatment of morbid obesity. *J Am Coll Nutr*. 2002;21:365–371.

Overweight and Obesity: The Surgeon General's call to action to prevent and decrease overweight and obesity. Available at: http://www.surgeongeneral.gov/topics/obesity/. Accessed June 20, 2004.

Weight-control Information Network. Gastric Surgery for Severe Obesity. Available at: http://www.niddk.nih.gov/health/nutrit/pubs/gastric/gastricsurgery.htm. Accessed June 20, 2004.

Organizations

American Society for Bariatric Surgery. (352) 331-4900. Available at http://www.asbs.org. Accessed June 20, 2004.

American Obesity Association. (800) 98-OBESE. Available at http://www.obesity.org. Accessed June 20, 2004.

The Bariatric Nutrition Dietitians' Discussion Group. To join the discussion, go to http://groups.yahoo.com/ or http://health.groups.yahoo.com/group/BariatricNutritionDietitians/. Accessed June 20, 2004.

Bariatric Surgery Clinical Research Consortium (RFA). Available at: http://www.niddk.nih.gov/fund/crfo/may2002council/rfac502_1.htm. Accessed June 20, 2004.